D0939029

SECRETS OF THE CANCER-SLAYING SUPER MAN

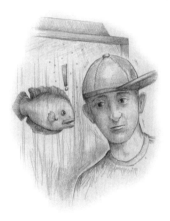

by Benjamin Rubenstein

Illustrated by Kenneth F. Raniere

Bethlehem, Pennsylvania: 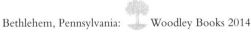 Woodley Books 2014

Cataloguing in Publication Data
Rubenstein, Benjamin 1983-
Secrets of The Cancer-Slaying Super Man:
The Story of a Boy and His Invisible Cape

Summary: A high school student survives cancer;
is hit again as a college student and beats it the second time.
His belief in his super powers helps him through
the grueling treatments and debilitating disease.
1. Benjamin Rubenstein 1983-   – Health Juvenile Literature
2. Tumors in children – Patients – United States–Biography–
Juvenile Literature [1. Rubenstein, Benjamin 1983-]
2. Cancer Patients 3. Children's Writings]
1. Raniere, Kenneth F., ill. II. Title
616.99'400924   978-0-9786472-3-0

Manufactured by Thomson-Shore, Dexter, MI (USA); RMA593MS060, February, 2014

For my parents and brother, who emptied
far too many puke buckets to count.

TABLE

OF CONTENTS

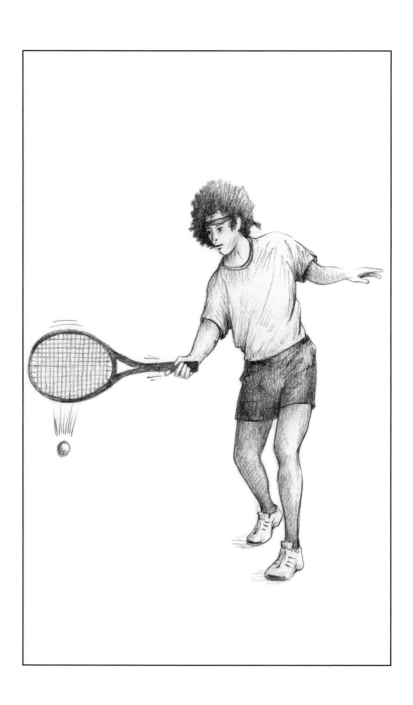

CHAPTER 1

The Wrong Kind of Super Power

If I could be stuck at one age, then I would choose to stay sixteen forever. The only drawbacks were not being able to get into an R-rated movie, and the hip thing.

On my sixteenth birthday I hopped in my car. For the first time, I was alone. I filled the twelve-disc CD changer with my all-time favorites. The freedom that came with being sixteen was a powerful thing. I was no longer just a kid. I no longer needed a ride to hang out with my friends. Though I didn't have a girlfriend – I was keeping an eye on Lily McGrath – I did have quite a few friends, like Andy Hardin, with whom I played a lot of video games. My oldest friend, from birth, was Drew Thornton, but Andy was the one I watched R-rated movies with. I had pals at school, too, including Bently, Nick Linebaugh and Worm. I was sixteen without a care in the world, except how to seduce Lily without having to talk to her.

The hip thing was a sharp pain, deep inside my hip, so deep that my mind couldn't pinpoint where it came from. The pain was simultaneous with my left Adidas's contact with the court. I pushed through the pain because the tennis season had just begun, and I wanted to make varsity. When I drove home that evening, my hip throbbed. It got worse. A week later, running became torturous. By the summer, I noticed a bruise and bulge in my lower back. Within weeks, I felt pain climbing steps. Then I could barely walk at all.

I called my brother Jonathan at Virginia Tech and he encouraged me to tell my parents about my pain. I wanted to wait until after our family vacation to Israel. Our summer vacations usually consisted of amusement parks, boring museums and the beach. I couldn't ruin this one.

Our tour group met in Jerusalem. We walked down Ben Yehuda Street with all the shops. I bought a white t-shirt with the Superman shield wearing a black top hat and Hasidic earlocks that read "Super-Jew." The shirt stayed in my drawer, collecting powers. When we climbed Masada, most of the group took the lift up to the top of the mountain. I decided to walk with Jonathan in the 115-degree heat. "Are you sure you want to do this?" Jonathan said. "It'll be hard, even for me."

"No way am I sitting this one out."

After the forty-five minute climb, though, I felt a pain that even Cal Ripken, Jr., would respect me for pushing aside. "When we get home I'll see the doctor and get it fixed. It's probably just a stress fracture," I promised Jonathan.

The day of my appointment, the surgeon had me stand facing away from him, and he pushed my pelvic bone for a minute. Just say it's a stress fracture, I thought as he prodded my hip.

"Something is definitely growing there," he said.

As we were driving home, I asked my mom, "What is it?"

"I'll tell you at home."

"What does 'growing' mean?"

"Please, Benjamin. I have to concentrate on this traffic. We'll talk about it at home."

That drive was the longest twenty minutes of my life. The word "cancer" entered my mind, but it scrolled too fast through my brain to register. She dropped me off in front and went to park. I waited at the kitchen table for her. My leg twitched. She gave it to me straight: "Benjamin, you have a tumor."

Boom! Her statement split my life into two distinct phases. Phase I was Pre-Cancer Ben: my first sixteen years, eight months, fourteen days and sixteen hours of life. Phase II began with, "You have a tumor," and will end when I die. After a long pause she said, "Are you all right?"

"Yeah, I'm fine," I said. Tumors are for Sick Kids. I'll never be fine again, I thought to myself.

"No, you're not. I can see you're not fine."

"I'm going downstairs."

I was on the brink of tears. I called Drew. "Dude,"

I said in a choked voice, "I have something to tell you."

"What is it?"

"I have a tumor."

"Oh my God, I think I just pooped myself."

In case it was a false alarm, I told Drew to stay quiet. "I don't want to make a big deal out of it if it's nothing." I don't know why I went to school the next day. I had been rocked by a life-altering uppercut. After school I cried for the first time in years. I went all-out but after a couple minutes I felt awkward and vowed never to cry again. I had not cried the day before when Mom said I had a tumor, so why cry today or ever again?

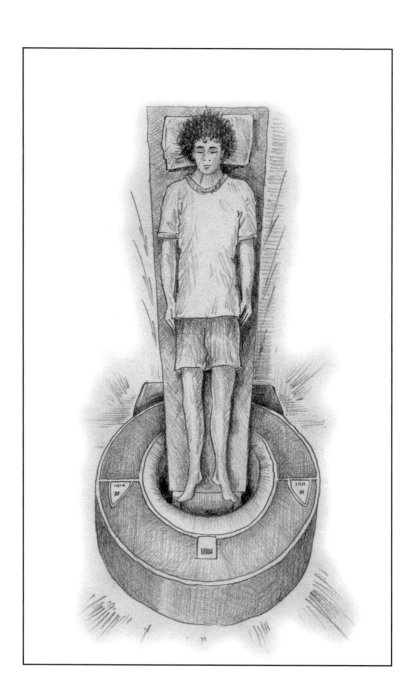

Chapter 2

New Galaxy at NIH

My parents and I drove over to the National Institutes of Health (NIH) in Bethesda, Maryland, during a school day for the first examination. We gathered around a large, round table. "You have Ewing's sarcoma, a rare bone cancer mostly found in teenage boys," Dr. Springs, the first of the NIH doctors told me. The tumor was located in my iliac crest and right next to the family jewels. The cancer, the disease, was alive, flourishing, invading my pelvic area, growing unabated right there.

Three days later, I climbed on the table in front of the cylindrical CT scanner. That three-minute scan of my lungs would reveal the probability of my survival. No spot, I would probably live. A spot and I would probably die. That's how my parents and close relatives saw it.

Me, I didn't even know what a CT scan was. I just held my breath like the robotic voice said.

The CT scan was one of the eighteen tests I underwent the week before treatment began. The other patients called it "Hell Week." There were two reasons for all those tests: to make sure I was healthy enough for what was to come, and to create a baseline for the rest of my life. Some of the tests were down-right scary.

One was apheresis, a procedure to try to create my own tumor vaccine. I would sit for five hours while my blood circulated from one arm to the other and a certain component collected. How bad could it be watching movies for five hours?

"But what if I have to pee? I asked the nurse as she stuck the IV in my left arm.

"Don't worry about that, Ben. You can use a plastic urinal." She wrapped the tourniquet around my right arm and cleaned the spot with alcohol. I turned away as she threaded the needle through my skin and up my vein. "Uh-oh," she said. Blood was streaming down

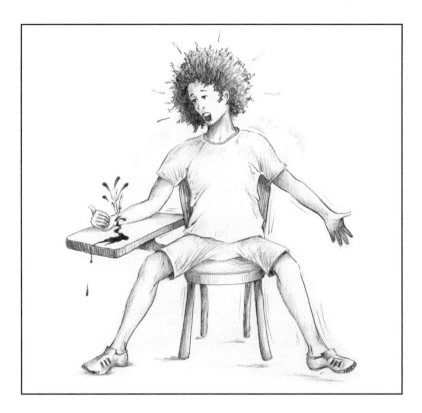

my forearm. My pulse sped up. My head pounded.
I was sweating, dizzy and nauseous.

I screamed at the nurse, "Take it out! Take it out!"
She called Dr. Springs down to console me. He said
that people often panic during apheresis. It wasn't true
but he was being kind. I had turned into a nutcase
because of some blood. If I couldn't handle apheresis,
then how would I handle chemotherapy?

SECRETS

At school I became certain that the girls no longer saw me as the shy, quiet guy who drove his friends everywhere and made the occasional quip. I was convinced they saw me as a Sick Kid. I know this because that is how I would have viewed anyone else with cancer. I would do everything in my power to show them otherwise.

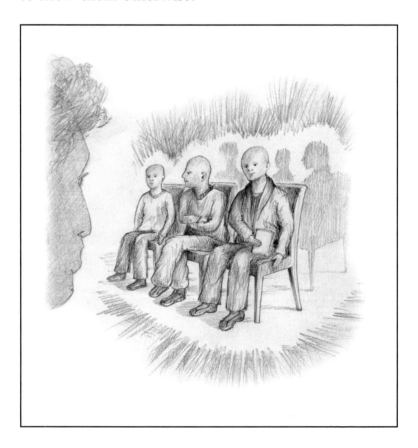

By September, I was watching a flurry of doctors at NIH. This behemoth hospital is only forty miles north of my parents' house but a galaxy away from anything I had experienced before. I was treated on the pediatric floor where the staff was playful with the patients despite how messed up they were. My primary nurse was Lisa Patrick, whom other patients nicknamed Pocahontas because of her Native American background. She was, of all the people in this strange new world, my favorite. She enjoyed teasing me for being quiet and always greeting her with a dull "hey" in my deepest voice. She called me a wuss if I winced when she drew my blood. I don't wince anymore.

The other patients were pale and completely hairless. They were people I wanted nothing to do with, because I never thought I would be a Sick Kid. The reality was difficult to deny in a room full of teenagers whom I would soon resemble. I was a Sick Kid. In the eyes of other people, I would never be able to discard the Sick Kid label.

SECRETS

Most were younger than me but there were two guys, Charlie Fletcher and Matt Cole, who were a few years older. Charlie had been in the Army stationed in South Carolina and Matt was a mechanic for the Army in Georgia. Matt and Charlie were so lively, wild and crazy, that I removed their Sick Kid labels.

In the hospital, I tried ignoring all the Sick Kids. Your life stinks, I silently said to them. "Mine doesn't. Just because we both have cancer doesn't mean we share anything else in common," I would think to myself. I wonder if subconsciously I did see myself as sick. Maybe I even still do, but I expect that thought will stay buried forever.

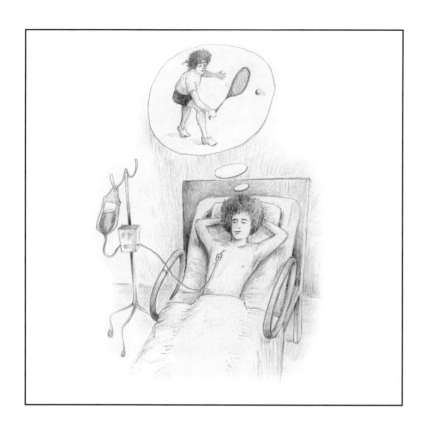

Chapter 3

Chemo Is a Piece of Cake

My small room at NIH had one bathroom. A blue curtain separated my bed from my roommate's. We each had a tiny television that we could rotate around our beds. I watched my favorite comedies without asking my roommate's preferences.

SECRETS

Opposite each bed was a small cot. One of my parents stayed with me every night I was there; nearly every second, in fact. They probably thought that I always wanted or needed them, but really they annoyed me by waking me, tugging my IV line, investigating my bags of medicine and asking questions. They responded to doctors and nurses for me, not by my request. They chatted with all the patients, even ones I wanted nothing to do with. They, not I, triple-checked IV bags to ensure all the information was correct. I was laid-back before treatment and I was going to stay that way. Cancer wasn't going to change that about me.

Chemo is a poisonous fluid that gets circulated around the body through a plastic port surgically inserted in the chest. A tube then runs through a giant vein and stops at the heart. This way the chemicals that destroy fast-growing cancer cells could be sent straight to my blood-pumper, without the hassle of first traveling through a peripheral vein. The port resembled a large bump on my chest and was proof that I had cancer.

Each day that went by without chemotherapy reduced my probability of survival, as if there were a percentage timer that continuously ticked down, ten-thousandths of a percent at a time. The teeter-totter of life levels off at the fifty percent mark, and then tips over until eventually there's a 500-pound wrestler sitting across from you and you're dying.

One of the worst aspects of cancer is fearing what's next. Fearing the unknown. Once I had experienced each part of the routine, like the chemo, I was no longer scared. It was like having an injury that causes pain – you learn to live with it, so long as it doesn't worsen. And when the pain does get worse, you adjust to that and say the same thing.

My first day of chemo was easy. My anti-nausea drugs knocked me out. When I woke up, my chemo was already completed, and I watched television and then went to sleep so the next day could begin.

No matter how cheerful I sounded, simply mentioning the subject of my troubles was an act of complaining to me. That's a standard I maintain.

SECRETS

Looking back, I may have been fooling myself into thinking that certain normal human emotions didn't apply to me. I don't know that my never mentioning cancer allowed others to misinterpret how sick I was. I never shared what my days were like, how important milestones were, or the cancer itself. But certainly that strong, silent outlook aided in my feeling of invincibility. All those other cancer patients complained about how hard it was, but I never once did.

The Saturday I was discharged from the hospital, I felt moderate pain around my tumor, which I envisioned as the cancer cells dying. I told them, "I am the ruthless destroyer of evil. You thought you could survive? I killed you in less than three days."

When I got home, I realized I was falling behind in my classes but I couldn't focus, even on a vocabulary worksheet. Cancer consumed me, and I couldn't get over how my life weeks earlier had been superior to my life now. What a difference one cancer day can have on your spirits!

I called Worm, a lifelong friend, to come over

and watch the Redskins game. I was the one who liberated him from his given name, Ethan Worman, to the cool "Worm." But before the game began, I got nauseous and rushed to the bathroom to puke. It looked like gallons of pink chunks, with some hamburger on the side. "Are you done yet?" Worm yelled. "That was disgusting. I could hear you all the way down the hall!"

The vomit was my emotional release. Once I barfed, my mood became giddy. Maybe cancer wasn't so tough after all. I rejoined Worm to watch the Skins win in overtime. From Worm that afternoon, I learned there were some things that not even cancer could change, like my friends, sense of humor and love for the Redskins. "I can do this," I said to myself. "One cycle down, thirteen to go."

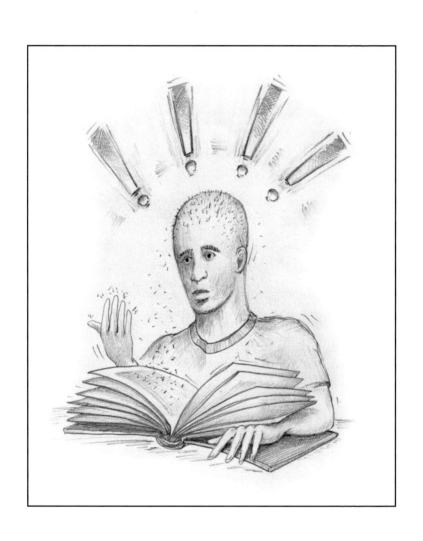

Chapter 4

Super Hairlessness

My hair began popping out and it wouldn't be long before I lost it all. My curly hair clung to my pillow, stayed in the shower drain and stuck between the keys of the piano. I had always kept a short tapered cut but as a sophomore, I let my hair loose and grew long, natural corkscrew locks. The girls at my school wanted to touch it, including Andrea Buchman who wrote in my yearbook, "It's been a great year. My favorite part is when I get to come in class to play with your wonderful hair. I swear I'm in love with it. I love you too, so don't get jealous. Have a good summer!"

Worm was envious and wrote, "Get a haircut!" Now I asked the barber for a close buzz cut to ease my anxiety when it fell out completely. He trimmed away.

SECRETS

I looked in the mirror and was frightened. "That's not me," I thought.

I avoided all cameras that year. I wasn't even photographed for the yearbook. Someone snapped a Polaroid of me with those therapy dogs people bring to hospitals. I ripped it in half. For a long time after the haircut I was scared of the mirror, scared of my silhouette. How could others recognize me when I couldn't recognize myself?

I was reading on the floor one afternoon when my head itched. I scratched and brought my hand down to my book in horror—hundreds of tiny hairs engulfed my fingertips. I wiped them on the carpet and rubbed my scalp. Again, hundreds of hairs. They were detaching like foliage on a windy autumn day. I rubbed my head under the bathtub faucet, peeling off clumps with each swipe. The remaining hairs fell out over the next day. I was as cancer-looking as it gets.

But it didn't look bad and even evoked some compliments. My friend Terry commented, "You have a nicely-shaped head."

"Yeah, sure."

"No, I'm serious. Some bald people have weird lumps on their head, but not you." As if my hairlessness wasn't enough, I needed help pooping. The only bowel movements I had taken over the last week consisted of small, hard balls, which I called nuggets. When I arrived at NIH for a biweekly checkup, I grabbed SpaghettiOs off the lunch cart.

"You shouldn't eat those SpaghettiOs," Charlie said. "That tomato sauce is brutal."

"He's right," Matt added. "You better be aware of your bowel condition. Sometimes, I have to go so bad that I'm running to the bathroom every five seconds. Other times, I'm afraid to go because it feels like I'm crapping a brick." A cancer patient's bowel condition represents his relative health. We may have had massive tumors, but if our constipation was under control, then we were fine.

When I visited Christine Pinot, my nurse practitioner and medical guardian, she listened to my belly. It wasn't making any sounds, so she said, "I think you might be constipated." To help push things through, Christine gave me the laxative milk of magnesia. I then sat in the waiting room.

I still wasn't pooping, but I sure felt like crap. My mom sat with me, reading her book, like a dog owner patiently waiting for her poodle to do his business. My mom had brought me magazines, but I was afraid to move my arm to turn the page.

You could have set a watch to my stomach cramps. As the minutes ticked away, they worsened. Yet the first few pooping attempts failed. Every time I exited the bathroom, my mom stared at me with a "How did you do?" expression, like I was three years old and learning to go potty. I shook my head and slouched back in my chair.

After several hours, I felt an excruciating abdominal pain. I rushed to the bathroom, swung the stall door open and flung the seat down. I temporarily blacked out from the agony. I looked at my masterpiece. Milk of magnesia had done the trick.

From then on as a precaution I drank the stool-softener Colace, up to four times a day. For motivation, I composed a short jingle:

> *Time for me to drink my Colace, it tastes so good.*
> *I have gotta drink my Colace, I bet you wish you could!*

Coming to a radio near you! To tame the beast, Christina prescribed mineral oil twice a day in addition to the foul-tasting Colace. The grossest thing about mineral oil was the end result − I pooped out the oil intact.

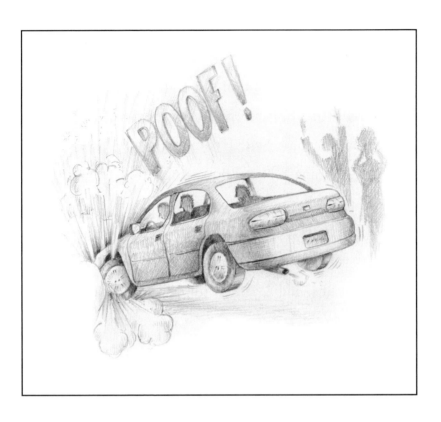

Chapter 5

Two Jokesters

You would think that life in a cancer clinic would be pretty dull but it wasn't – as long as Matt and Charlie were there. I had met Charlie on my first visit to NIH, overwhelmed and virtually mute. Charlie had cajoled me until he managed to get a laugh out of me.

SECRETS

Charlie had suffered for months at an Army hospital in South Carolina losing seventy pounds. First he was diagnosed with shin splints and then with compartment syndrome, where compressed nerves damage muscle and impede blood flow. Both diagnoses were bogus, so his mother enlisted their Congressman to intervene. Once Charlie was transferred to private care, he was diagnosed with bone cancer. The physician was amazed at how big Charlie's tumor was. Because of the treatment delay, his cancer had already invaded his lymphatic system. His surgeon recommended amputation, but Charlie convinced him to salvage his leg in what must have been an impossible decision. After surgery, he received a radiation dosage that left his flesh crispy-charred black. He began walking again two weeks after his surgery and throughout radiation. He might have had a few super powers himself.

Matt had been a mechanic in the Army when the docs diagnosed him with pneumonia, without even taking an X-ray. Then he lost sensation in his shoulder and arm, and now the docs said it was pneumonia plus a bug bite. When Matt vomited blood, the docs finally took X-rays which showed tumors. They evacuated him to Walter Reed hospital, and then to NIH.

When in the treatment room together, Matt and I would find humor in our preposterous cancer stories. We debated whether constipation was preferential to diarrhea, and agreed that NIH should have stocked an abundance of baby wipes. We discussed how he'd have to learn to throw a baseball with his left arm since cancer had taken his ribs and his right lung.

Matt and Charlie would compete. When Lisa told them to hydrate, they would guzzle water until they felt sick. Matt's ability to down a liter within seconds always propelled him to victory. When Charlie's leg surgery went thirteen-and-a-half hours, Matt begged his surgeon to prolong *his* to fourteen hours. The surgeon said he could not go over six hours, so Matt negotiated to keep a piece of his cancerous rib in a jar. He carried that rib around like a trophy.

A cancer-surviving friend of theirs who had his leg amputated in childhood climbed a rock wall and challenged Matt to follow. Matt pointed out his recent shoulder surgery and inability to use his arm. Charlie harassed Matt until he climbed that wall with his good arm and chin. Matt then went swimming in the ocean and Charlie sat on the beach where he arranged everyone's prosthetics into a comfy beach chair and table arrangement, packing the legs with ice and using them as cup holders. They then spent the next two weeks in-patient together, isolated with infections and on antibiotics. Matt and Charlie had unique ideas on how to cure cancer, like drink alcohol until the tumors were saturated, or thread electrical wire into them.

One boy on the floor had cancer that caused him to go blind just before getting his driver's permit, a source of immense frustration to him. On Christmas Day, when the NIH parking lot was deserted, Matt and Charlie took this blind boy out for his first drive. The car lunged, jerked, sped, spun doughnuts and occasionally hit snow banks. Blues Brothers music blared out the open windows while Matt and Charlie shouted directions, laughing wildly.

"When I finish chemo, I'm going back to upstate New York. I'm going to drink beer and go fishing every day. I can't wait," Matt told me before finishing treatment. Matt and Charlie didn't take life too seriously. They took midnight post-chemo trips to Krispy Kreme, packing the car with anyone willing to join them, and ordered dozens of dough-nuts each. They then drove back to NIH and puked Krispy Kremes all night.

Matt called his artificial rib cage his "Auto Bondo Body," because the material was similar to the putty used in chassis repair. Not even Matt could rival Charlie's goofiness. Charlie once put his finger up his nostril during a scan. Then he frantically displayed the film to Lisa proclaiming a serious problem, who rushed it to the doctors. When the doctors reviewed the scan, they missed his prank entirely. Charlie finally explained what he had done, and as they caught on, they laughed as hard as he did. Lisa finally forgave him after a few days.

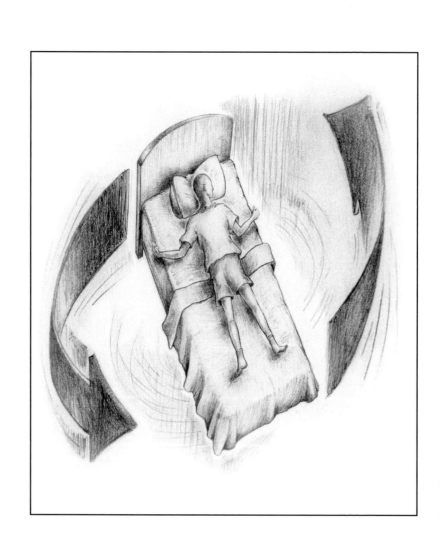

Chapter 6

Sports, the Cure-All

And so I went on with life as if nothing were wrong. It was just a little cancer, no big deal. My treatment followed a precise schedule: when the cycles began and ended, and when I could expect my white blood cells to fall and rise. All of my doctors had warned me about neutropenia – when the white blood cell count drops dangerously low – which could lead to a serious, possibly fatal infection, because the immune system no longer has the ability to fight. Neutropenia can last for several days beginning a week after each cycle of chemo. When you become neutropenic you try avoiding infection by washing your hands and staying away from people. This is an aspect of the cancer world that most people don't know about. Neutropenia is no joke.

SECRETS

My doctors warned me the tenth day from the beginning of each cycle could be the worst. After showering on that tenth day I stepped over the tub and reached for my towel. The room began to spin. I glimpsed the mirror and my eyes rested on the disgusting bump in my chest. My figure was blurry, full of dark spots. I began shivering and became nauseous. My right ear started ringing, and I could hear my heartbeat. This must be death.

I assumed I was about to pass out, so I yanked on my boxers, scurried to my room, and sprawled out on my bed. I was experiencing acute symptoms of anemia, another side effect of chemo. Once I lay down, the symptoms vanished.

While neutropenic, I took my temperature every two hours. When the thermometer showed 100.4 degrees, the temperature that doctors consider feverish, my parents rushed me to NIH. The NIH doctors had conditioned the word association "neutropenia," "terror." Never mind that a temperature of 100.4 poses no immediate danger, or that neutropenic fevers can be flukes that don't amount to actual infections, or that I felt physically fine. That was a fear I never, ever want to experience again.

We arrived to a calm hospital staff and not the frantic one I had expected. The nurse directed me to a regular hospital room devoid of intensive care equipment. Dr. Springs looked me over, noting the acne that had spread across my back was worse than J.J. Redick's.

After Dr. Springs left, I switched on the playoff baseball game between the New York Mets and San Francisco Giants. I ate a grilled chicken sub, forgetting that I had no appetite. That day was a turning point in my treatment and understanding of cancer. It is necessary for doctors to implant fear in patients. But as I clarified what could and could not kill me – and why – I felt less like I was stricken with cancer, and more like I was surviving cancer.

Watching that game in the safety of the room at NIH made me realize everything was going to be okay. My parents were keeping an eye on my vital signs. The docs knew the numbers. They understood the risk.

SECRETS

I had been so terrified of neutropenia and the accompanying potential for death that I figured I would be too messed-up to even watch the end of this baseball game. Instead, I saw Benny Agbayani crush a home run to catapult the Mets to a 3-2 victory. Who would have thought a baseball game between two teams I don't care about would be so impactful?

Sports were part of my regular routine. I watched all the baseball playoffs, every televised NFL game, and critiqued every Redskins game. The NFL kept my life moving. Each Sunday that passed meant that another cancer week was gone.

After a few hours, my dad walked me down to radiology for a chest X-ray. Every patient who was admitted for neutropenia received one as a precaution, along with vancomycin, an antibiotic. We got to talking about the Yankees, and how, even if you hate them, it's hard not to respect some of their players' postseason performances. Through 1999, Derek Jeter batted .326 in the playoffs. During that same time period, Mariano Rivera's ERA was a staggering 0.38

with thirteen saves. Rivera hadn't given up a single run in eighteen consecutive postseason appearances, including six World Series games. He may be the best postseason pitcher ever. It was sweet to have something on my mind besides death.

Man, I needed something to hold on to during that first month of cancer treatment. With Jeter and Rivera, the Yankees weren't going anywhere until they would beat the Mets in the World Series on October 26. I adopted the Yankees as my team, sharing them with my dad.

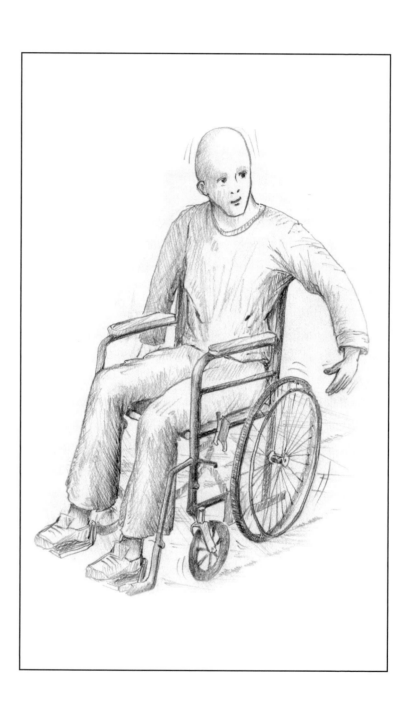

Chapter 7

Chicks Dig the Car

The Make-A-Wish Foundation grants wishes to children with life-threatening illnesses. Many young kids want to meet stars or athletes. I wanted a car.

"I don't think you can get a car," the hospital social worker said after I inquired. "But you can get a lawnmower. They won't get you anything that goes over ten miles per hour."

When I had gotten home from the hospital after Cycle Two, I talked to my friend Andy about my wish. "I could try to get a guest spot on an episode of *Friends*."

"No way, this is what you should do…have them get you a private dancer."

"I'm sure *that* would fly with my parents. You know they have to sign off on this."

"Tell them you need it for your cancer. Tell them to get a second dancer for me."

Without restrictions I would have wished for the Batmobile. With the ability to reach 350 miles per hour with afterburner thrust, I would never be late to anything again. And I would always have a hot girl with me when I arrived.

I narrowed my wish down to playing flag football at FedEx Field with friends and some players from the Washington Redskins, and going to Super Bowl XXXV in Tampa, Florida. Then I had my epiphany: I'd wish for an entertainment system worthy of being on *MTV Cribs.* My parents received a letter in November saying "It is our desire that a wish fulfilled will provide your son with hope, strength and joy as he fights his illness." I didn't know about all that, but I did know it would make my sitting time much more pleasing.

In December, my Make-A-Wish Foundation toys arrived, including a fifty-three inch high-definition television. The TV was bigger than the shelf, so my parents hired a carpenter to build a new platform. I was watching sports and Jessica Alba in high definition before most people knew what HD was.

I brought Andy down to the basement to see the system. "I think your TV is bigger than my living room!" he said.

"I know it is."

"Look at you, you're gloating. You showed me the TV just to brag, didn't you?"

"No, of course not."

"Why don't you open up the blinds to get some natural light in here?"

"The instructions for the TV say that you can't let sunlight hit it."

"You're such a dork."

"Don't hate just because you're jealous."

My delight was halted because, similar to my feeling lousy on the tenth day of Cycle One, I woke up on the tenth day of Cycle Two unable to move without becoming light-headed. Painful sores, called mucositis, infested my mouth. Mouth sores are a

common side effect of chemo and occur from a break-
down of the tissue lining the mouth. My body couldn't
repair the sores until my white blood cells increased.

By late morning my temperature reached 100.5, so
my mom drove me to NIH. I could barely walk to the
elevator. I almost always refused the wheelchair–
except this time. I believe that if I can stand, then I can
walk. Most people would call my condition "being
sick." I called it, "messed-up." Even years later, my
friends make references to when I was sick. I correct
them. "Don't you mean when I was 'messed-up?'"
"Messed-up" made me feel strong. Rather than feeling sick, I saw a normal teenager who happened to be
receiving deadly poisonous drugs to fight off the round
cells that were attacking his body.

While I watched college football at NIH that night,
I tried eating a hamburger. Each bite blazed; the two
sores on the side of my mouth and the one under my
tongue inhibited my eating, drinking and talking. Dr.
Springs found a solution to my mouth pain. "I have a
topical anesthetic that might do the trick," he said.

"I tried it out earlier to make sure it works."

A few days after being discharged, I returned
to NIH for scans to see what my tumor was doing.
It had shrunk substantially, proving the chemo was
effective. I expected nothing less. It was *my* tumor,
and I had never lost a battle yet. In a lot of cancer
books, you read about acceptance of the disease, and
death. They acknowledge that the cancer might kill
them. These survivors say they felt like they could
do anything; that the world was in their grasp. They
say their fears vanished, like their fear of rejection
or saying something stupid. They could live in the
moment, carefree, having already faced death, having
nothing to lose. I realize now that by not fearing my
demise, I missed out on something special, something unique to survivors, a feeling that cannot be
manufactured.

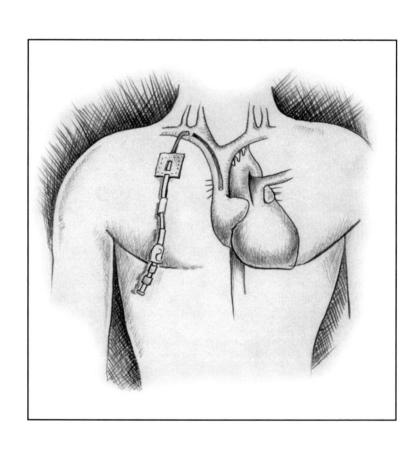

Chapter 8

Vampire Treatment

I would receive fourteen cycles of chemo, including eight long cycles consisting of five infusion days and six short cycles with only two days of chemo. Cycle Three was my first long cycle. The morning after the last day of chemo, I woke up ready to go home, but I needed a blood transfusion. Before I started cancer treatment, my mom read an article claiming that the American Red Cross failed to screen some blood. After that, she wouldn't allow me to receive any stranger's blood, but instead had volunteers drive to NIH to donate. Statistics show that direct donations are no safer.

Blood donations have a forty-two day shelf life, after which they are discarded. Direct donations – drawn for a specific person – could not be used for anybody else. My mom claims she planned the donations perfectly, but it was impossible to predict exactly when I would need a transfusion. My home-room teacher, Mr. Foley, claims that I'm one-third his because I have gotten so much of his blood. Maybe if I got Tom Brady's blood, I would be playing quarter-back and marrying a Brazilian supermodel.

I watched the thick red liquid creep down the IV tube. Once out of sight, I lifted my shirt and stared as it entered the giant needle in my chest. I wanted to know the exact second it hit my bloodstream. My blood transfusion took longer than expected, so it was six o'clock when I was discharged. My nurse pulled the huge needle out of my chest and covered the bleeding hole with a Band-Aid. I darted out of bed and rushed my mom out the door. The blood energized me, like a vampire. I was furious that I had to stay there so late, my legs wobbled from disuse and I was famished.

"Let's get out of here and go to McDonald's," I said. My mom considered my idea of eating greasy McDonald's so soon after receiving chemo awful, but I insisted. The ride home lasted just over an hour. It felt like eternity. I could see nuggets and fries, and sundaes, oh my. My mouth watered with the thought of a succulent burger. We passed two McDonald's en route to my favorite one.

I shouted at the drive-through speaker, "I'll have the Double Quarter Pounder with cheese Extra Value Meal, with a Coke. No mustard." I had never eaten a double DQP, but there was no better time to try it than now. I demolished the fries by the time we got home and then ate most of the burger. I didn't vomit or get nauseous. If this had been a short cycle, I would have thrown up a kidney. I also did not become neutropenic. My immune system stayed normal, as if it was barely affected. I once said to Lisa, "Have you noticed that I don't become neutropenic for long cycles?"

"Yeah, Ben, that's really amazing."

"Have you ever seen that before? Everybody else seems to."

"No, I can't recall that happening. Some people get neutropenic but don't get a fever. That's pretty common for the long cycle."

SECRETS

I had super bone marrow, and word got around.
Several months later, another patient finished treatment
and headed home to Florida. During our good-byes, he
gave me something "I saw this in the store and thought
of you," he said handing me Superman boxers and a
blue Superman t-shirt. Now my Super-Jew shirt has
something to play with. "You have earned it," he said.
I was flattered that my fellow cancer patients noticed
my powerful super marrow was superior to anyone
else's. Matt always joked about how easy treatment was
for me compared to everyone else. "You breeze right
through this stuff," he said. I saw my resilient bone
marrow as a sign that I was supremely capable of
battling cancer. I possessed something extremely
unique, and I reveled in it. I was better than the other
patients, better than everyone, better than humankind.
The next obstacle to tackle was my surgery, and how
bad could that be? After all I was The One. I was a
Super Man.

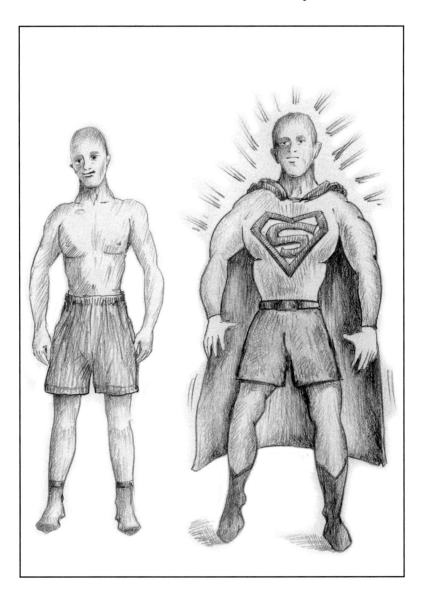

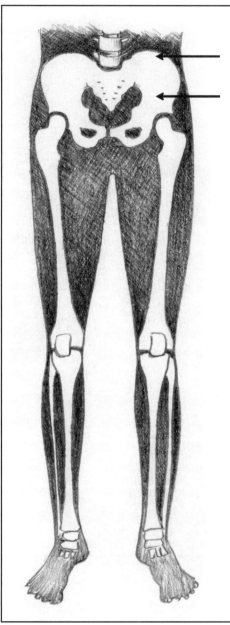

The tumor has shrunk substantially on the iliac crest of the pelvis.

Iliac wing of the pelvis.

Chapter 9

The Wonder Hip

My surgery was going to be so early that we decided to stay in Washington D.C. at my aunt's house overnight because it was closer to the hospital. At six in the evening, we left. Goodbye, house. I had to leave my sweetheart flat screen behind. When we arrived at my aunt's, Jonathan and I watched *Erin Brockovich*, which sucked, and I fell asleep halfway through it, half-dreaming:

"What will it feel like to see your little brother all messed up tomorrow?" I dreamed I asked.

"What will it feel like to *be* all messed-up?" he fired back.

"I don't know. At least I'll be asleep. I won't even know what I look like, but you'll have the image forever. Every time you talk to me or look at me you'll be reminded."

"Maybe, so long as you pull through."

"I love you, big brother. You know that, right?"

"Yeah. I love you, too."

It only happened in my head but that's what we could have said, or should have said.

The next morning a nurse threaded the IV and gave me a mild sedative. My heart pounded so loudly I thought it might explode through my chest. My life would soon be in the hands of professionals for several hours. Some serious surgery was about to transpire: cutting, sawing, stitching, stapling and bleeding. I didn't want to lose the use of my leg; or lose my life.

The nurse eased the bed through the double doors into a large room. I glanced right and saw my surgeon, Dr. Merlin, preparing instruments. In the middle stood a bed surrounded by tables with silvery tools displayed on them. Everything was there except a chainsaw. "Why don't you slide over to the other bed and dangle your feet over the side?" the nurse suggested.

"Okay. What are you doing?"

"I'm going to put in the epidural now."

"Is it going to hurt?"

"Just a pinch."

"Don't worry, Benjamin," my mom said. "I'm here."

"Are you ready?"

"Yeah…that wasn't so bad."

"Hold still so I can secure it…there we go."

"Am I going to need an enema?" I asked.

"No," the nurse replied.

"Good."

"Benjamin, I have to go now," my mom said quietly. "Don't worry, you'll be okay. I love you."

"I love you, too."

"He'll be just fine."

The anesthesiologist said, "What I want you to do is slide your feet onto the bed, and push back a bit… good. Now, lie down on your back. Don't worry about the needle, that's secured."

"How's that?" I asked.

"Good."

"Can you tell me before the anesthesia starts so I know when I'm going to sleep?"

"Of course. Now, just relax."

I looked up at the ceiling with three nurses and the anesthesiologist staring down at me. It was like something out of a movie. Then boom, somebody turned off the lights. I woke up in the recovery room a mess: my left leg was in traction with a large bandage around my hip, my eyes were covered with ointment, a small suction tube was inserted through my nose that went down the back of my throat and into my stomach, an epidural was in my back, three epineurals were feeding pain medication into my nerves. I had oxygen tubes in both nostrils, a catheter was coming out of my penis, two IVs stuck into my right arm, two more IVs into my left arm and a large breathing tube was shoved down my throat. When I noticed the breathing tube, I freaked and began to choke on it.

I have almost no recollection of what happened next: I couldn't speak or move anything except my finger, so I tapped my mom's hand. She called over the anesthesiologist.

"I think he wants the breathing tube out."

"I can't take it out yet, he just woke up. I'll take it out in a short while."

"Are you sure, because I think he really wants it out."

"I can only remove the tube if he holds his head up for ten seconds." I heard him loud and clear. I lifted my head above the pillow and held it suspended as tears streamed down my face.

"Okay, I'll remove the tube," the anesthesiologist said.

I will always remember the screaming around me that day: the dude next to me whining about his leg pain, the girl to my other side screaming as she came out of brain surgery. No amount of opiates in the world could stop her pain. Dr. Merlin told us the surgery had gone well. He asked me to move my foot from side to side and wiggle my toes. "Oh, I'm so glad to see him do that," my mom said.

"Me too!" Dr. Merlin said.

I asked my mom how many blood transfusions I had received. "We had thirteen people donate for you. You got all of that blood, and still needed one more.

SECRETS

Since Jonathan hadn't donated, we sent him down. He was the fourteenth donor." The volume of blood in fourteen transfusions is more than my body holds, meaning I lost all my pre-surgery blood plus some. I just hoped my dad's blood would not infect me with his love of salmon.

Despite what I told him, I wanted Jonathan to come home with me after surgery. At the time I thought I needed him there. If I was this helpless in a hospital, I didn't know how I would manage being at home without him. Would Mom and Dad be able to take care of me by themselves? Would I be able to handle the loneliness? I wasn't about to slow him down by asking him to give up his life for mine. But I had seen how cancer stalled the lives of some of the other guys on the floor, like Charlie and Matt. They were away from home for so long getting treatment that I wondered if their old lives would still be there if they could survive and get back to them.

A year after my surgery, I asked my surgeon to send me digital pictures of the operation, and reluctantly,

I looked at them. I was split open and the skin was folded down on itself. There were pools of blood and multiple tubes coming in and out. I could see the bone and it was colored blue, either because of dye or the cancer cells. I was unrecognizable, even to myself.

I'm just glad that nobody photographed me after the surgery. I have an idea of what I looked like then, but it's nice to not have that visual image as a constant reminder. Other people still have the image of me as a Sick Kid, but I spared myself.

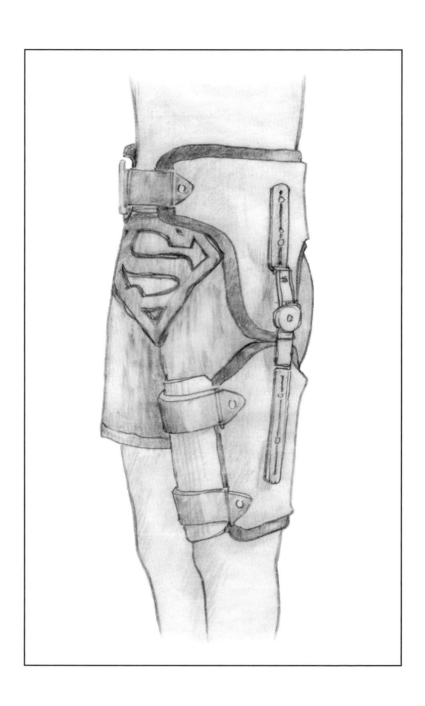

Chapter 10

Booting Cancer's Cheeks

My first day back to school after being absent for three and a half months felt strange. Many friends celebrated my return, but nobody did it like Bently. He sprinted through the cafeteria with a big poster of two butt cheeks labeled "Cancer," and a boot kicking them labeled "Benjy." The top read, "Welcome Back. Way To Kick Cancer's Butt." With only six cycles of chemo left, I remember thinking, "I can see the end of the road. I'm almost there."

I had been using crutches to allow my hip to heal, but at my ten-week post-surgical checkup, Dr. Merlin said, "Stop using your brace and start bearing weight on your leg. To do that, take a partial step as you're crutching. It'll hurt at first, so start with just putting thirty pounds down."

"If I accidentally step with more than thirty pounds, will it damage anything?" I said.

"No, it's just going to hurt."

"What happens if I fall? Will that do any damage?"

"No, you can fall right now if you want proof."

When I got home, I ripped off the brace and tossed it into the closet. I collapsed on my La-Z-Boy and stretched back feeling total freedom. It took time to conquer the fear of stepping with my left leg. Sometimes I would forget to limit the weight I put on it, and just like the surgeon said, it hurt.

To celebrate this milestone, Drew and Worm took me to Hooters, for the wings of course. After, we went back to my house. I decided to enter through the front door—even though there were seven steps to the front porch— instead of my usual route through the garage. My dad saw us coming, so he opened the front door and walked outside.

"Hey, boys. Benjy, why aren't you entering through the garage?"

"I have to learn how to go up steps someday, right?"

Without realizing that my left foot had not yet cleared the final step, I tumbled. My dad caught me before I hit the ground and helped me up. I felt foolish, and wished my dad hadn't seen me fall. He blamed Drew and Worm.

"Don't worry about it. That was my fault," I explained to them once we got inside. "My dad's just scared that I hurt myself."

"Yeah, we know," Drew said.

My parents loved that my friends came over. "You're lucky to have such good friends," they told me as they provided a constant supply of Ho Hos and Twinkies. At dinnertime, my parents invited my friends to stay for a meal. The truth is that we had a blast as we played games for hours each afternoon and evening.

A year later, I talked to Bently about those good old times. "If it hadn't been for you guys, I probably would have lost my mind. I really appreciate you hanging out with me so much."

Those were some of the best times of my life," Bently said. "When you were off getting your chemo, we didn't know what to do. It was so boring not playing PlayStation at your house."

Dr. Merlin played a different kind of game in which I was his star patient. As he tested my strength and mobility during my checkups, he would talk about me to his fellows in Doctor Speak. Dr. Merlin's confidence was contagious. He thought he was the best surgeon in the world, and the way I deconstructed his bragging to the other docs, he thought I was the best patient ever. I thought there should be a poster of me on his walls: Be the best patient you can be. Be like Ben Rubenstein. Dr. Merlin praised me, and for that, I loved him.

Nearly my entire left iliac wing was removed up to the joint, as well as part of my sacrum, and some muscles and tendons. My hip muscles were reattached to others in my abdomen, lower back and butt with dozens of staples and some tape. My scar is fifteen inches long and it took fifty staples to keep it closed. Without a bone to stop its migration, my femur — that's the thigh bone — shifted up, causing my left leg to be higher off the ground than my right leg.

My body has compensated. Forces normally sent through my hip have been transferred elsewhere. My gait has changed. This bothers me, and to this day, I still try to walk straighter. All these years later, Dr. Merlin says it's amazing that I can still walk pain-free.

My hip was quirky:

• I felt knee pain referred from my hip anytime my knee was elevated above my hip joint.

• The entire left side of my left leg was completely numb. I now have some sensation.

• I could feel either staples or bone fragments under my skin near my hip flexors.

• When I rubbed the left side of my lower back, I felt it in my penis.

• My left leg would never be nearly as strong as my right.

• When I stood on both legs to pee, the stream stuttered. I usually stand with my left heel slightly raised, like a dog.

• I will always have an obvious limp.

• I will never run or jump again, though don't dare challenge me in darts or bocce.

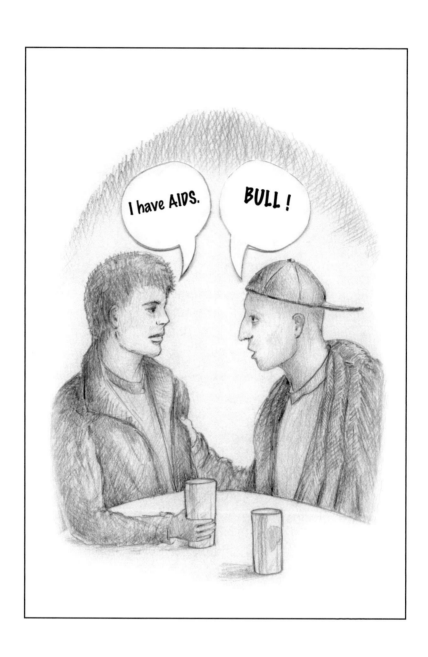

Chapter 11

My Friend and His Invisible Cape

My physical therapist, Kevin Linde, was short and Jewish like me, so we immediately hit it off. We could always talk about sports, video games and fast cars. I progressed with Kevin's help, and would have strengthened even faster if it had not been for the chemo cycles and neutropenia.

"Every time I move forward I have to break for chemo," I complained.

"I guess I'll just have to push you harder when you get back," Kevin said.

Because I limited the weight on my left leg, I walked on the handrail platform at physical therapy. As the weeks passed, I braced myself less and less. This time, I raised both arms out to the side and stepped.

"Look!" I said for confirmation I wasn't hallucinating. No crutch, brace, or handrail – just normal walking.

"From now on, use one crutch," Kevin said. By the end of June, I ditched my crutch in favor of a cane, and by year's end I was walking unassisted. Months later, I would have nothing more to gain from physical therapy.

The spring of our senior year, Bently and I skipped our last two classes to see *Spider-Man* the day it opened. We left our calculus homework assignments with Nick to submit for us. I attached a note to our teacher that would read: "I had to go see *Spider-Man*. Please don't punish me. Actually, today is my last day of physical therapy. After fifteen-and-a-half months, I'm finally done." I finished the note with a smiley face.

Nick and I became close back when I was still getting chemo and physical therapy. He was Catholic, yet probably possessed more Judaism knowledge than I did. Because Nick had hemophilia, a bleeding disorder, I felt like he understood my trial more than my other friends. He was the only person I talked to about my disease.

Nick picked me up two weeks after finishing Cycle Seven to eat lunch at Taco Bell. "I have something kind of important to tell you," he said on the way.

"I already know…you have a small penis."

"No, it's a little more serious than that." I already knew Nick was a hemophiliac. How much worse could it be? My heart skipped a beat.

"I have AIDS."

"Bull," I snapped back, wishing he were lying.

"No, I'm serious."

"I know you are." I steadied myself. "How did that happen?"

"When I was a baby, I was on a hemophilia medicine composed of blood products. At the time nobody really knew how to screen blood, so my medicine was contaminated with HIV. By the time I was seven years old I had full-blown AIDS."

"Wow." I was silent for a moment, thinking. "How'd your family deal with it?"

"It was weird at first, but it's cool now. Nobody babies me."

"That's good. So I'm the first friend you have told, huh? What an honor. I'm glad you told me, but why?"

"I don't know. Sometimes I just feel like talking about it, you know? My dad used to tell me to keep it to myself, that nobody else had a right to know. But recently my dad's been feeling differently. He even encouraged me to tell you."

"I feel bad that I'm the only one who knows. Our friends give me props for taking on cancer, but you have been living with AIDS most of your life. If you don't share what's going on, you won't get the respect you deserve."

"It doesn't matter to me. You deserve all the props; I respect what you're going through."

"How do you prevent your family from pitying you?"

"They don't pity me. They admire me for my hardship. My mom's a nurse, remember? You and I are the same—we don't need any pity."

Nick and I jabbered about our diseases through lunch and on the ride home. When I asked Nick which disease he would rather have, he said, "People generally will take what they have because they're scared of everything else. But knowing how much AIDS sucks, I think I would rather have your cancer." I agreed with him. Cancer can be killed. AIDS is a lifelong disease with no cure. I bet Nick would give anything for an AIDS cure, even one as virulent as chemotherapy. It is a miracle he has lived this long. Maybe Nick had super powers he hadn't told me about. After that, Nick and I had many conversations about life that lasted until the sun came up.

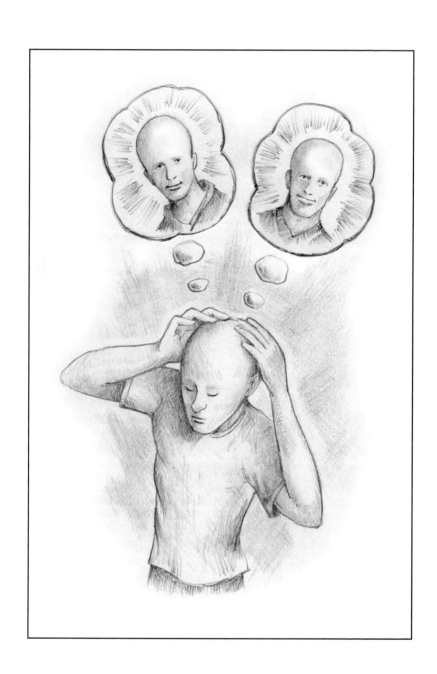

Chapter 12

Still and Always Two Jokesters

Finally, in early August, I watched the last drop of chemo enter my bloodstream. After ten months of allowing the most toxic liquid any human voluntarily injects into his or her body, I was done. My nurse threw my last empty bag into the biohazard receptacle. That's it, no more chemo ever again. The nurses presented me with a banner they signed that read, "Congratulations Ben!" I didn't want them to ever forget that I was the teenage patient who physically and psychologically annihilated bone cancer to an extent they'd never before seen. In my mind, ending chemo was going to be an accomplishment worthy of a Diddy yacht party, but when it actually happened, it was a big nothing. I had to begin radiotherapy just three days later.

And then my mom dropped yacht-sized news on me. "I just got off the phone…Matt passed away four days ago."

"What? That's not possible; he finished treatment months ago and was doing so well. What happened?"

"He developed an infection in his artificial rib cage and went in for surgery, but then developed a large blood clot. NIH is having a memorial service for him this Sunday."

Now, despite my intention of being invincible, I struggled withholding tears. I rushed to my room so that Mom couldn't see me shaken. I had considered Matt a friend, yet I barely knew him because my Super Man complex prevented me from opening up to other Sick Kids.

I could not feel like most people. Sometimes I felt hollow, like the title character from my favorite show, *Dexter*. Trauma as a little boy made Dexter into a psychopathic serial killer – "a monster," he calls himself. Dexter kills out of need. Dexter questions whether he can change into the person he was supposed to be had the trauma not occurred. In the end, he can't. A monster is who he is.

My need to withhold emotions factored into the creation of my Super Man complex. I shut down feelings to endure cancer. But denying any emotional response was like eating cherry Twizzlers: once I started, I couldn't stop. I eliminated fear and sadness from my consciousness. I came as close as any sane guy can get to thinking he can deflect bullets. Imitating Superman boosted my self-esteem. Feeling invincible fed my ego. The more deluded I became about my super powers, the more I could cope with the inconveniences of cancer. Like Superman himself, I became detached, the resident of another world.

Unlike Dexter, I never consciously decided to be that way. I didn't get to consider if I was better off as a Super Man. A Super Man was who I was now.

Dexter is unable to reach out to people close to him out of fear that he'll hurt them. I couldn't reach out for fear of being seen as the Sick Kid. I needed people to see me as a Super Man. Dexter was empty by nature;

SECRETS

I had made myself hollow by a subconscious force. The shrinks call this an attachment disorder. I call it a survival technique. With Matt dead, I worked overtime to keep my feelings for him from flowing out.

Matt had driven down from upstate New York the day before his surgery to correct the infection in his Auto Bondo Body. He stayed with Charlie and coughed all night. Charlie pounded his back trying to dismantle the congestion. Just before his operation, Matt told his doc he didn't feel well and closed his eyes. Charlie waited as the doc frantically tried to save him. Then he sat with Matt until he passed.

I saw Charlie at Matt's memorial service and he didn't look well. We talked about PlayStation 2, and then I went home. I had a policy of not staying in touch with other cancer patients, so I didn't know that Charlie's cancer had never gone in remission. That was the last time I saw Charlie. As with Matt, it was only after his death that I could admit I cherished him.

With Matt gone, Charlie lost the will to fight. He had been through so much. At the end of his life, his

mother told me, Charlie mostly slept while a constant parade of friends and family visited. The night
he passed, he sat up and pointed to the door, and said,
"Matt's here!" He then drew his last breath.

"Charlie and Matt are probably up there cracking
jokes about us right now," Charlie's mother said at his
memorial service. Others struggled in the wake of his
death. I wasn't part of that: my identity as a Super Man
had prevented me from getting close to other cancer
patients, even if they were as cool as Matt and Charlie.

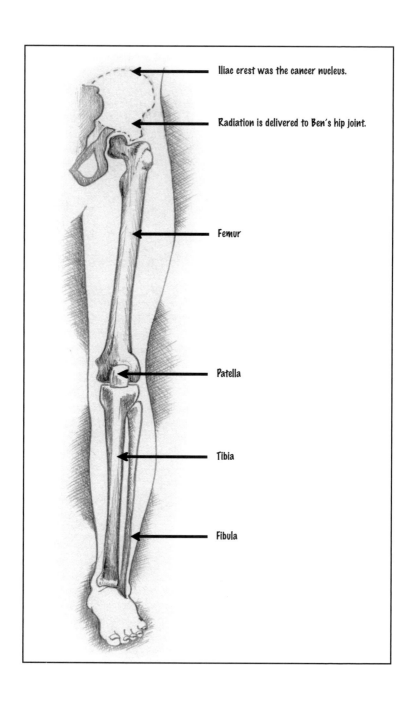

Iliac crest was the cancer nucleus.

Radiation is delivered to Ben's hip joint.

Femur

Patella

Tibia

Fibula

Chapter 13

Me, It's What's for Dinner

While walking around our cul-de-sac on a cloudy, cool day Jonathan came out saying, "Benjamin, you might want to go inside. Mom is going crazy."

"What?"

"She keeps screaming that you're not wearing sunscreen and the sun is dangerous."

"I have been outside for five minutes."

"I know, she's crazy. She has just lost it."

I knew I had to be careful, but five minutes could certainly do little harm. I may not have tanned in the summer of 2001, but I sure got cooked. In order to leave my hip joint intact, my surgeon, Dr. Merlin, had not been able to remove the bone margins that have been proven most effective to completely excise the tumor. For that reason, I needed radiotherapy.

SECRETS

Christine explained the concept of margins to me: "If you dropped a bucket of sand in the same spot, most of the particles would clump together, but some would fall away. Cancer cells aren't much different. Your iliac crest was the cancer nucleus, but there was no way to tell how far some of the individual cells had wandered."

Radiotherapy is a scary idea—beams of concentrated X-rays shooting through parts of your body at different angles. To ensure the radiation is delivered in the precise location each session, permanent tattoos are given to the patients. "Lie on the table and pull your pants down," the technician said. "Are you ready?"

"Yeah, go ahead."

She reared back and jammed what looked like a Bic pen into my skin six times. I received radiation every weekday for five consecutive weeks, totaling twenty-five sessions. When I arrived for my first radiation session, a nurse escorted me to the big microwave and positioned me where I remained motionless. I did not want those energy waves anywhere near places they didn't need to be. The nurse exited and closed the mammoth door behind her, leaving me all alone. The machine grumbled and I think it moved around. I couldn't see what was happening because I had buried my face in a pillow. I was supposed to be scared of radiation, but I never was. Marinate me, baby. I often napped as the beams mutilated my cells. Sometimes it felt warm, but that was all there was to it.

My radiation oncologist must have spent hours designing my treatment plan. He showed me the diagram he had made. Beams emitted from multiple angles, covering a large area from the top of my thigh to the bottom of my ribcage. My radiation dose was moderate – 4,500 rads – delivered to my hip joint, the remainder of my ilium and sacrum, the top of my femur, and part of my bowel. Different organs and tissues can tolerate varying amounts of radiation, which is why the radiation was dispersed. Radiation and chemo are amazing in the sense that they kill cancer and other cells that divide quickly. But, they can also create new cancers. I was given a five percent chance of developing a soft tissue tumor fifteen to twenty years later.

With radiation, my skin transformed to a red so bright that it frightened my friends. I had also developed diarrhea, which intensified to the atomic variety. Since it took over an hour to get home, I often pooped before leaving NIH – just in case.

I still had seven radiation sessions left when my senior year of high school began. My parents wanted me to get tutoring until radiation was complete, but I refused. By the end of the first week, I was exhausted, yet still determined to attend school. The following week I arrived at school early and met Bently in the lobby. "Dude, I only have two more radiation sessions, then I'm cancer-free."

"That's awesome," he said with a high five.

I officially became cancer-free on September 14, 2001 at approximately 3:40 p.m. – exactly one year after Phase II of my life began, almost to the minute. I had been waiting for this ever since Dr. Springs said to me, "You have Ewing's sarcoma." My cancer was in remission, and life could return to normal. I thought something dramatic might accompany the freedom from cancer, but nothing really changed. My left iliac wing didn't suddenly grow back, and the months lost at NIH were gone forever. Having cancer was similar to not having cancer – they were both part of the gradual path known as my life.

Events occur, milestones are reached, and life just keeps moving along. Even though I was surprised at what a big nothing becoming a survivor is, my family made a big deal about it. My mom bothered me until I agreed to celebrate at Pizza Hut, which I called the "Cancer Ravaging Celebration Dinner," or CRCD. My aunt sent me a $50 gift certificate to Outback Steakhouse for finishing treatment. I saved it for a special occasion, like taking Jessica Alba on a date. I ended up using it for my first anniversary of surviving cancer because Jessica had never returned my calls. I was glad that my relatives made a fuss because secretly, I wanted CRCD to be a national holiday with a parade down Pennsylvania Avenue where I would stand next to President Bush on a float, smiling and waving to the hordes of excited supporters.

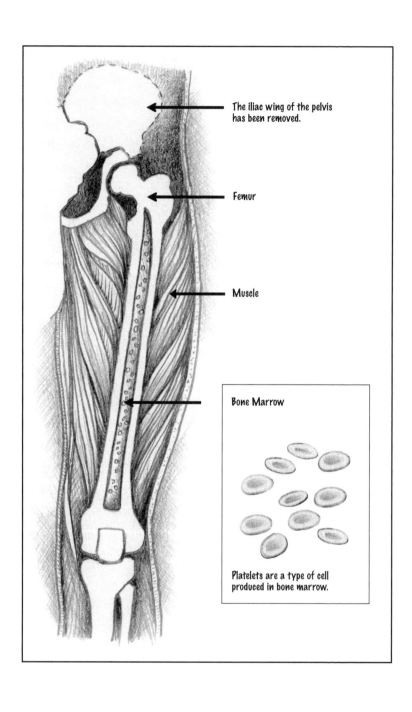

The iliac wing of the pelvis has been removed.

Femur

Muscle

Bone Marrow

Platelets are a type of cell produced in bone marrow.

Chapter 14

Lightning Strikes Again

I needed to get away from home and was glad that college was coming up. I applied for early admission to the University of Virginia. UVA wait-listed me. Then in mid-June I received that delicate piece of mail from UVA, possibly making me the last student accepted.

My freshman roommate Derek Miller was one of the few people who seemed interested in my past. After I mentioned my Make-A-Wish gift, he said, "You should bring your TV to school. It would take up our entire room, but it would be worth it. I'm willing to sleep on the hallway floor."

I didn't acclimate to college well. I barely made new friends or talked to girls, vomited from too much alcohol, and wished I could get in fights without causing hip damage. I refused to sacrifice exercising, sleeping or watching TV for studies. Did I even belong at UVA? I looked forward to the semester ending and being back home with old friends. Winter break was like old times. I spent many nights at Brent Birdsall's house. Birdsall and I discussed my eighteen-month post-treatment checkup, scheduled for the following day.

"What kind of appointment do you have tomorrow?" Birdsall asked.

"It's nothing, just a standard visit."

"I pray for you every time you go to the doctor. I cried when you told me you got cancer."

"Are you serious? Man, even I didn't cry. Thanks, but I don't need the prayers. I'm doing really well." I said this because everyone commented on how healthy I looked, how well I was doing. I felt just as strong as I did when I was sixteen.

I was disappointed to learn that Lisa no longer worked as a nurse in the pediatric cancer unit, but had moved to Research on the same floor. I guessed that she could no longer cope with the sadness of getting to know Sick Kids, only to watch them suffer and die.

Back when I was getting treatment, Lisa had asked me if I wanted to be a doctor when I grew up. "Are you going into medicine? Or maybe try to cure cancer?"

"Yeah, right. Once I finish treatment, I'm going to walk away and never look back at this or any other hospital."

Christine was nonchalant during my physical exam. Before leaving, I asked if my blood results were available.

"I don't think so, but let me check." Fifteen seconds and several mouse clicks later, Christine said with a surprised tone, "They have you red-flagged."

"What does 'red-flagged' mean?"

"Your platelets are dangerously low at 24 thousand." Platelets are a type of cell produced in the bone marrow that assists in clotting. Boom! My bone marrow was dying without my even knowing it. IMPOSSIBLE. The words "bone marrow transplant" flashed in my head like a lightning storm. I knew Round II had begun, and my life was about to change again.

"24 thousand? Oh, my God. Normally, I'm way over 200 thousand. What is causing my low platelets? Am I going to need a bone marrow transplant?" I asked.

"That would be a long ways down the road because we don't know the cause. There are many possibilities. It could be nothing, or a disease," Christine said.

At home, my mom asked how things went, and I provided the sugar-coated version. Still, seeing her face as she said, "Oh dear God," broke my heart. She called Christine.

"What did she tell you?" I asked.

"She said that lightning doesn't strike twice, and so the chances of this being leukemia are small."

I had assumed my bone marrow was failing. It hadn't occurred to me that this might actually be cancer again. That suggestion made me dizzy and seasick, like my couch dropped from under me.

I returned to UVA following winter break. The next day I woke up hearing myself shouting, "Get me a tissue!"

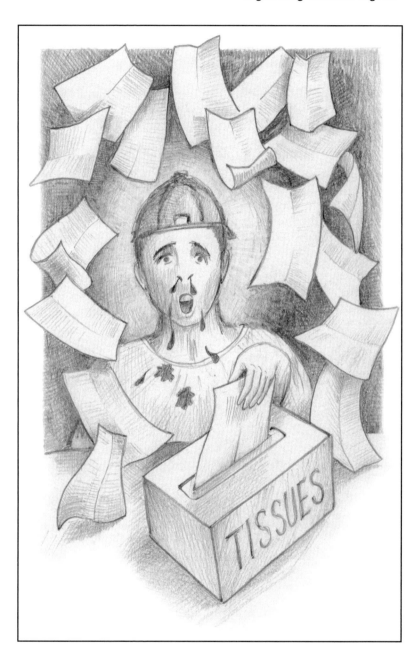

SECRETS

"Whoa man, you got a lot of blood there," Derek said. I had felt an itch on my nose upon waking. I suppressed it with my navy blue pillowcase, and looked over in horror as I saw red streaks. I began going through tissues like toilet paper after eating bad Chinese food. Each tissue was soaked in blood, and there was no stopping the downpour. I called NIH and asked to speak with the doctor on call. "Hey Ben, this is Dr. Springs."

"How's it going, Dr. Springs? I was lying here when suddenly my nose started bleeding."

"How fast is the blood coming out?"

"Pretty fast. I'm mowing through my box of tissues."

"Okay. Go to the ER. I'm going to call them so they know you're coming."

As I hung up, Derek was standing in the doorway holding my keys. "Benjy, you ready to go?" My bleeding finally slowed while I was in the waiting room. A nurse took me to a patient room and inserted an IV to take blood.

"The results will take an hour. Then we'll get

you some platelets." My platelet transfusion couldn't
come soon enough—the blood loss from my nose
was replaced by an IV. I had just finished cleaning up
when Derek returned from parking.

"Hey bud, did the bleeding stop yet?"

"Almost. She just took my blood, so it'll take an
hour before I get the results. You can head back if you
want."

"Nah, that's alright. If I go back, then I have to do
work. I'd much rather just watch TV here."

"Thanks, man."

When I first met Derek I didn't like him much
and had trouble getting used to his quirks.

Over time, he grew on me. After that day, I
considered Derek my good friend.

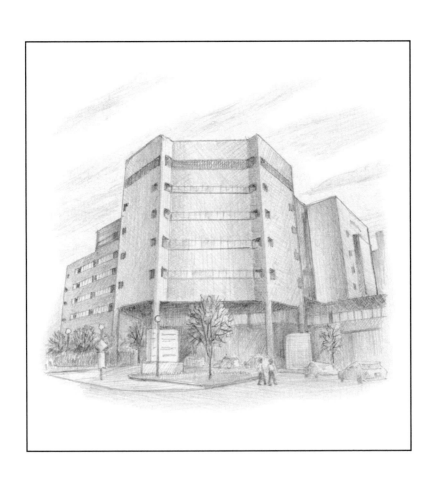

Chapter 15

Chemo's Gift and Curse

My bone marrow was dying so fast it was scary. Within weeks of discovering there was a problem, I was already receiving blood and platelet transfusions regularly. NIH did not possess the technology to diagnose my problem, so Christine referred me to Johns Hopkins Hospital for a bone marrow biopsy.

Weeks later my family and I met with Dr. Ford, head of the adult bone marrow transplant program at Hopkins. He shared my diagnosis: I had myelodysplasia, an acquired genetic abnormality of the bone marrow in which the seventh chromosome had mutated. It was almost certainly caused by the Cytoxan chemotherapy I received for Ewing's sarcoma. Ironically, that would also be the cure: I needed a bone marrow transplant or else myelodysplasia would develop into leukemia.

I asked for the survival rate. Without hesitating Dr. Ford said, "The universal number is thirty percent." Thirty percent chance of living. Seventy percent chance of dying. My heart skipped a few beats.

I needed a second opinion, so Christine arranged a meeting with Dr. Bruce, a pediatric oncologist at NIH with a great knowledge of transplants. "The University of Minnesota offers a fairly new form of transplantation using stem cells from umbilical cords instead of from the actual bone marrow," Dr. Bruce told me.

"Okay, then. I've narrowed my treatment center choices down to Hopkins or Minnesota."

During our flight to Minneapolis, I turned around and saw my dad staring out the window with a curious look on his face. "Benjy, let me show you something... look out the window and at the wing. Do you see?"

"See what?"

"The wing is flapping around out there!"

"It's supposed to do that," I said.

"No, I don't think so. That wing is flapping because it's going to fall off!"

Chemo's Gift and Curse

As we descended towards Minneapolis–St. Paul International Airport, I saw hundreds of frozen bodies of water, one after another. The sky was gray and looked like it could start snowing at any second. I knew that once I stepped out of the airport, I would feel the cold, crisp air of the Midwest and watch as my breath formed a cloud, a pure sign of my existence.

After several mild winters, Virginia had been pounded by a blizzard in February that left us with eighteen inches of snow. That was when I first discovered there is something about those crystalline snowflakes dropping from the sky that makes me feel alive. Cancer had given me a newfound esteem for every season and condition, including heavy rain. "Who likes rainy days?" Derek once asked me.

"I do. I like the smell of the rain. It smells peaceful."

The Minneapolis airport was monstrous. When we finally reached the exit and I walked through the automatic doors, my eyes watered with the temperature plunge. I took a deep breath and smiled because it felt good. Bracing.

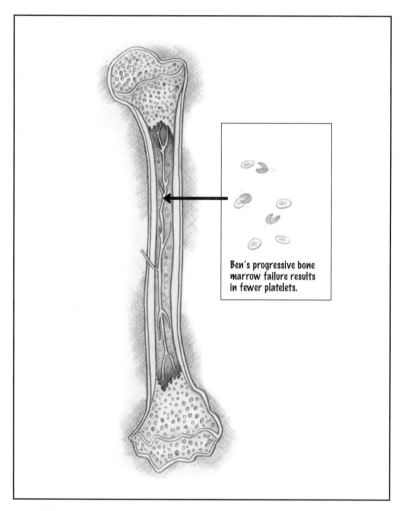

Ben's progressive bone marrow failure results in fewer platelets.

We had come to the pediatric transplant clinic to meet Dr. Fry to learn about umbilical cord stem cell transplants. In 1990, the University of Minnesota had performed the first cord blood transplant for leukemia. Its biggest advantage was the low incidence of graft vs. host disease, or GVHD, one of the most severe complications of a transplant. Stage One GVHD is good because it shows that the new marrow is active. Stage Three is severe and Stage Four is life-threatening.

Even if the recipient developed GVHD, the severity would be less than that of a traditional transplant. There were proportionally fewer cases of Stage Three or Four GVHD with cord blood transplants and many fewer deaths. It took less time to find a cord blood donor because the match didn't have to be as perfect. Dr. Fry was reluctant to provide me a survival figure, but I got it out of him, hoping his would be higher than Dr. Ford's. "It's about forty percent for full blown leukemia and sixty percent for myelodysplasia for a patient who has not had previous chemo. Because of your previous cancer treatment I'd put you at fifty percent." Half the patients live—it was clear as day I would be one of them. Now we just had to wait for a match to turn up.

Back at UVA, the transfusions kept my hemoglobin and platelets at manageable levels, and I had no other side

effects. I didn't feel sick, tired or weak. I felt fantastic.
However, at three in the afternoon one day, I couldn't
wait to leave. I was waiting patiently in the lobby, listening
to 3 Doors Down, when my nurse tapped my shoulder
and said, "Ben, your mom is on the phone."

"Listen, I just got a call from Minnesota…they have
found a match and want to know whether you'd prefer
to start in one week or two," my mom said.

"They already found a bone marrow match?"

"Isn't that great?" she said.

"Yeah, I guess. Already?"

"Dr. Fry wasn't lying when he said cord blood finds
a match quicker."

"So, what do they want to know?"

"They have to schedule you, and need to know if
you want to start in one week or two weeks."

"No point in staying around here any more. I guess
just a week."

And just like that I left my home for a new one
halfway across the country where the unusually amiable
natives speak with an odd accent, and my closest friend

was a thousand miles away. The first test performed at the clinic was a blood draw, more fittingly described as a blood drain. I was forced to watch a video on bone marrow transplantation and sign a consent form, which contained the word "fatal" six times. This was no Hell Week. I was entering Hell Months. My dad joined me the next day in the OR for my bone marrow biopsy and spinal tap, which were performed just to be certain that I still had zero leukemic cells.

I was neutropenic. Just three months after being red-flagged for low platelets, my rapid cancer had already destroyed nearly every blood cell in my body. It was difficult to accept that my bone marrow, the core of my Super Man complex, was self-destructing. On the other hand, I did comprehend that my chances of survival were limited and then I had to convince myself that they did not apply to me, because I was Super Man. "Complain all you want," I told this cancer of mine. "Soon you'll be dead, Myelodysplasia."

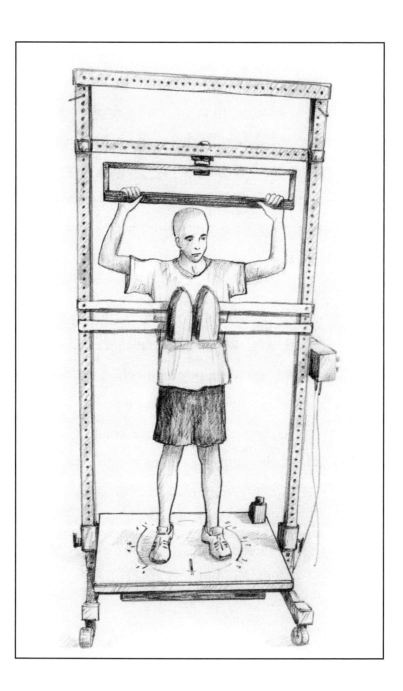

Chapter 16

The Cord of Life

I awoke after surgery in my new home on the fourth floor at University of Minnesota Medical Center, with a picturesque view of the Mississippi River a hundred yards away. I had just had my Hickman catheter surgically implanted in my chest. A Hickman is much like a port—the difference is that the Hickman catheter protrudes out of the skin, and then separates into two different IV lines, allowing simultaneous drug infusion.

Before receiving my transplant I would need three days of chemo and four days of radiation in order to completely eliminate my bone marrow. This conditioning regimen would create a ticking time bomb with no known time of detonation. For the following weeks, my germfree room and countless blood and platelet transfusions would be the only things to stall the explosion.

I would undoubtedly die if the transplant hadn't come along to save me. I couldn't believe I was getting chemo again just eighteen months after Cycle Fourteen's final bag was tossed into the biohazard receptacle. When the chemo was complete, I felt grateful that it only had lasted for three days rather than ten months. After a respite from treatment on the Sabbath, my nurse woke me up.

"Time for radiation. There's a man here to escort you." As part of my conditioning regimen, I would receive total body irradiation that would blanket me, no escape. I would absorb 1,350 rads over four days, with two sessions each day. The technician manufactured lead blocks so that my lungs only sustained partial radiation.

I stood motionless with my arms elevated for five minutes, and then faced the wall behind me for five more. My hairs stood on end and a wave of nausea burst through my stomach. I wanted to close my eyes, but then again, what was the point? Instead I stared into the big, black eye of the machine. When the second set of five minutes was complete, the technician sent me back upstairs.

Some of my nurses were gorgeous, especially Jen Albright, who made me tingle inside and red in the face. I maintained a crush on her for the next two years. On Transplant Day in late morning, Jen brought in a pathetically small bag of red liquid. I did a double take. This is supposed to save my life? Before Jen released the valve so the stem cells could flow through my veins, she asked, "Is there anything you would like to say first?"

I longed to say the *Shema,* a Jewish prayer, but instead said, "Do your job, little fella."

My *No Complaining* rule prohibited me from being dramatic. It was no joke, and I knew that. Jen released the valve and the stem cells swarmed into my Hickman. Now, there was only one thing left to do—pray that my baby donor, whom I would never meet and whose name I'll never know, had the right kind of cells to give me a third chance at life.

Generally speaking, I was in a constant feverish state, which was fairly normal but still taken seriously.

SECRETS

My new marrow repopulated very slowly, leaving my immune system open to virtually every disease. Fevers could be caused by GVHD, infection or my body's response to the growth of new bone marrow. The brightest transplant doctors in the world with access to the best technology can't always determine the cause.

For a month, my doctors had been saying I would be released soon. But every time my departure seemed possible, a complication would develop. I was permitted to venture outside and take a walk, or sit on one of the hospital benches, but I declined. My mom couldn't understand why. Perhaps cancer's greatest gift is the perception that when human desire is left unfulfilled for long stretches of time and then is finally satisfied, the joy proves to be worth the wait. I wanted the day I was released to be the sweetest redemption of all, and I didn't want to diminish it with pointless breaths of fresh air.

Thursday, June 19 was the day the docs said I could leave. My punishment had been sixty-five consecutive days in the hospital, so my reward of

freedom would be great. I had forgotten what the
world looked like without peering through glass. My
mom and I rode the elevator down, walked past the
hospital lobby and through the automatic doors. A
revolving door and five feet stood between me and
the world. I paused to consider my accomplishment.

I did not breeze through my transplant the way I
had tolerated my Ewing's treatment. Now I understood
what other Sick Kids had gone through, how making
it to the other side can be a struggle, a tug-of-war with
not only cancer, but also with hope.

I entered the revolving door, pushed it all the way
around and stepped onto the concrete outside. It was
a warm afternoon with gray, low-
hanging clouds smothering the sun.
A calm breeze touched my face. I
lifted my particulate mask off and
pulled in a slow, deep breath. The
leaves had never looked greener,
and the world had never looked

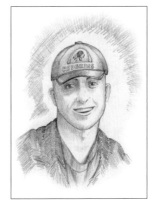

clearer. This was the single happiest moment in my life.

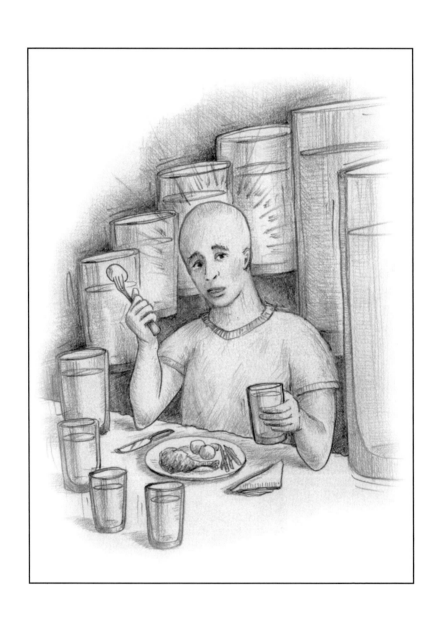

Chapter 17

Bring Back That Sports Cure

After 122 days in Minnesota, I flew home for
follow-up treatment at NIH. NIH was directly associ-
ated with my cancer, one of my life's most significant
events, making it an equally important location to me.
NIH consumed my time, and not just hours or days,
but months. So many cancer patients spent their time
there. They were Sick Kids even though we shared
the same illness and appearance I did not consider
myself to be like them. NIH's rooms, structures and
some of the staff lacked human traits, like empathy,
and transposed them onto some of us. That helped me
feel, and even be, more like Superman. NIH helped
make me that way by fostering an atmosphere where
that feeling could grow, which created the code that I
lived by:

SECRETS

- Survive.
- Don't cry.
- Don't complain.
- Don't show pain.
- Don't show fear.
- Don't question your ability to survive.
- Don't question your superiority.
- Think of cancer as normal.
- Don't let cancer make you sad or jealous.

Not everyone could become as flawless as the cancer-slaying Super Man that I was at NIH when I had Ewing's sarcoma. But not even Superman could be Superman all the time. He had to put his time in as Clark Kent. At less than a hundred pounds, my cape was now hanging on by a thread. I felt like I was falling apart. I couldn't look in the mirror, like after my haircut three years earlier when my curly locks had fallen to the barber shop floor. My muscles were tiny and soft, nothing like the firm fibers I had developed weightlifting at college. My shoulders slouched with the weight of my head. A meteor storm of kryptonite

had assaulted me. I was fading into oblivion, and my
super powers could not stop it.

At my six-month post-transplant checkup, I had
a lip biopsy, one of the best determinants of GVHD.
I had been fearful of graft vs. host disease since my
transplant, but by this time I begged for it. My salivary
glands had stopped working. I had to chew my food
until it was mush. Even then I had to gulp water,
like I was taking a pill. My eyes were dirt dry, which
caused excessive tear production. The tears pooled
in the bottom of my eyelids until overflowing and
streaming down my cheeks. My lips shed thin layers
of yellow skin. My bowels switched between both
extremes. Since GVHD has its own treatment, I
figured that would make me healthy again. If it wasn't
GVHD, then I didn't know how I would continue
surviving. The following week, I received the phone call
from Dr. Fry that I had been anxiously awaiting. "Your
lip biopsy showed evidence of GVHD, so you're going
to start taking prednisone, a basic steroid."

SECRETS

I had never been so happy to have a life-threatening condition, because now I finally had a treatment that could fix me. I couldn't wait to begin my steroids. If they didn't work, then traditional ancient Chinese medicine was probably next. Bring on the bear bile and toad venom.

The most significant side effect of prednisone is bone thinning. A DEXA scan, which measures bone mineral density, showed that I had osteoporosis. A voice began screaming inside my head. No. That can't be. I'm only nineteen years old.

"You've received so much chemo and radiation that your bones can't produce enough new cells to keep up. There is medication that may reverse the effects and build more bone," my doctor said. I had accepted the bone cancer, that I had no left hip, and that I would never run or jump again. But now I struggled with believing that, at nineteen years old, my bones were shot.

I returned for therapy with my former physical therapist, Kevin Linde. Under Kevin's direction, I lifted weights because I believed a strong body would

offset what I was missing elsewhere. I lifted to prove
that I was still strong after surviving cancer twice. The
stronger I appeared, the less likely someone would
perceive me as the Sick Kid. My osteoporosis was later
downgraded to osteopenia, which is a milder loss of
bone mineral density.

When every organ seemed to be deteriorating,
and every muscle atrophying, and my life slipping
away, I became well. The cure wasn't an experimental
treatment or an invasive procedure, but the simple
steroid, prednisone, which gave back my life force.

I hadn't used the term Super Man as a joke. It was
my strengths in fighting cancer that led me to believe
I was a Super Man. No other term could describe my
extraordinary resilience to disease and my capacity to
survive the cure. Unlike my cancer-ridden left ilium,
my Super Man complex was the one thing I had that
no one could take away. Like the code I continue to
uphold, my faith in my super powers remained. My
invisible cape is still tied around my neck. No matter
how it seems I should feel about these amazing powers,

they will always be a part of me, even if they are nothing other but a remnant, like a single cancer cell that can't be killed, waiting for its time to flourish again.

During the first three months after prednisone restored my life, I was content with precisely what I had. Everything felt special, from going to my weekly checkups with Jonathan, to watching the evening edition of *SportsCenter*. I had never been happier over a stretch of time that long.

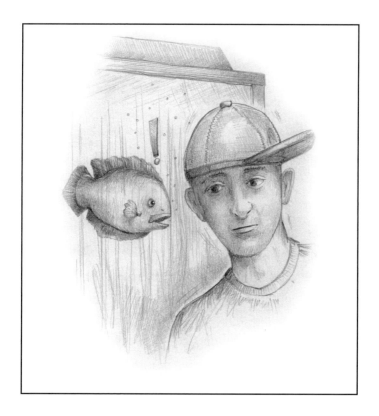

Chapter 18

Galaxies Conquered

The difference between me living with cancer
and me recovered from cancer comes from the little
things. Although I assured myself that I would never
again take anything for granted, that's impossible now
that I'm healthy. Riding in the car is just a car ride.

Listening to music is nothing more than that. Cancer gives everything meaning. The memories of Pre-Cancer Ben are just as persistent. I can't cruise with the windows down and the stereo blaring without remembering that first summer of driving freedom, before the cancer.

A doctor once told me, "It's a miracle you're alive, an absolute miracle. You may not even know how lucky you are."

I understand a little. I'm in my third chance at life. That may be all I have. I still uphold the *No Complaining* rule which, believe it or not, has value. People in good shape can find things to grumble about. People who are fighting for their lives don't have that luxury. For instance, I see myself in relation to Matt or Charlie, whose deaths act as reminders that they would give anything to be where I am today. They did give everything, but everything wasn't enough.

I am still, after all this time, averse to sorrow. I remember wanting to cry the day after I learned of my tumor. I considered how hard I should cry, and chose to sob. Right away, I felt awkward, so I regained control and vowed to never cry again.

And I haven't. After that cry, Super Ben was born. I decided that I was somehow special, not just in my ability to deal with cancer, but in all of life. I was convinced that there was something in me nobody else on earth had. I had never felt that way before cancer, which gave me the opportunity to see those cavalier feelings.

Since the first drop of chemo entered my bloodstream, many things have changed. I would probably be taller if I hadn't gotten cancer while I was still growing. I have many allergies. My eyes are too dry. My skin is too dry and itchy. My hemoglobin is too low. My red blood cells are too small. My heart beats too fast. My bones are too thin. My gallbladder is too stony. My intestinal blood vessels are too narrow. My kidneys are too stupid. My scars are too frequent. My hairs are too infrequent. My left testicle is too large. My left leg is too short. My bone marrow and blood type are no longer my own. My brain is full of knowledge it shouldn't contain. My eyes have witnessed disturbances they shouldn't have seen. Most importantly, my physical ability has been snatched from me. But I think throughout everything, my personality has held steady; I'm still patient, shy, generally happy and easily humored. I'm still me.

If I could do it all over again, go back to the tennis court and feel no pain, never learn the difference between a lymphocyte and a neutrophil, never receive an ounce of chemo and never have uncontrolled cell growth, would I do it?

I don't know the answer. If I say yes, I forfeit relationships with Derek, Kevin and countless others. Then again, I would gain my hip back. I would relinquish the extensive knowledge nurses and doctors instilled in me. But I would have two years of my life to be a high school student and college boy instead. It feels good not to have an answer because it gives me something to think about. I vividly remember what happened to me, whereas most of my friends look back on those years as a blur. By living through things that I was never prepared for, and having long periods of isolation where I had time to think about them, I have achieved a crystal clear vision of my past. I love having these memories be so clear. I don't think I could ever give up that clarity.

There was an ugly old fish in the NIH waiting room that always seemed to be watching us. What did he think as he swam around? Did he think the guy who sweat every time he got his blood drawn was funny the way I did? Did he notice the kid who ate the pasta salad his sister prepared for him no matter how bad he felt? Did that old fish smile when a girl used the word "cheemy" with her friends to make it sound more appealing?

It was a relief to finally be out of that fishbowl where visitors would sit around my bed, staring. I had felt so pathetic. I wanted to get up and walk around the room just to show them that I could. But I couldn't. I was hooked up to IVs and sentenced to stay. That world of my cancer brothers and sisters could still be mine if I weren't one of the fortunate ones. I never lose that world…but I left it behind.

RESOURCES FOR CHILDHOOD CANCER

NONFICTION
Armstrong, Lance. **It's Not About the Bike: My Journey Back to Life.** Despite the controversy, he is the most famous cancer survivor ever. Scribner, 2000.

Castro, Duane Bailey. **http://www.thejournalofaprizefighter.** A beautiful site about bridges on New York City's periphery by a cancer survivor. Since 2007, Duane has been cancer-free. He apprises readers of his progress with the disease and shares his breathtaking photographs. 2009.

Eggers, Dave. **A Heartbreaking Work of Staggering Genius.** Taking care of his kid brother after his parents die of cancer, the narrator captures the mood of survival. 2000.

Gaes, Jason with Adam Gaes; Tim Gaes. **My Book For Kids With Cansur.** A picture book imbued with hope from a young boy who later died of cancer. Melius & Peterson, 1987.

Jaouad, Suleika. NY Times blogger. **Life Interrupted: http://well.blogs.nytimes.com/author/suleika-jaouad/** A Lower East Side writer shares the experience of five days of chemotherapy. 2012.

Munroe, Randall. **http://xkcd.com/.** Some of his comics are about cancer, as his then-fiancé was diagnosed with breast cancer in 2011.

Piccolo, Brian. **A Short Season.** Football player who died at 26 after seven month battle with cancer shares his story in this classic autobiography. 1971.

Rosen, Michael. **Michael Rosen's Sad Book.** A personal account of grief over the loss of his son with various ways of dealing with the melancholy that attends it. "Sometimes sad is very big. It's everywhere. All over me." Candlewick, 2008.

Rubenstein, Benjamin. **Twice.** A boy's story of overcoming cancer two different times as a teenager, first as a high school student, then as a college student. In remission for a decade now, he is the funniest, smartest witness to both the disease and its cures. Woodley Books, 2010.

Schimmel, Robert. **Cancer on Five Dollars a Day (chemo not included).** Da Capo. Stand-up comedian Robert Schimmel's edgy, hilarious, and poignant musings on his battle with cancer. 1971.

Small, David. **Stitches: a memoir.** This graphic memoir is as much a movie as a tale of redemption that informs us that things can get better, that good can emerge from evil, and that art has the power to transform. W.W. Norton, 2009.

Sundquist, Josh. **Just Don't Fall.** In the end this is the story of a young man making his way in the universe and is thus a little rough around the edges. **Just Don't Fall** is a book that will encourage young men to stick to their goals even when the going gets rough and they have no strong mentors. Penguin, 2010.

FICTION
Dodd, Michael. **Oliver's Story: For 'Sibs' Of Kids With Cancer.** This picture book is aimed at explaining cancer to young children in the primary grades when their brothers and sisters get cancer. Candlelighters Childhood Cancer Foundation, 2004.

Honenberger, Sarah Collins. **Catcher, Caught.** In his own search for identity in the face of death and his parents' insistence on alternative treatments, the narrator follows in the footsteps of Holden Caulfield. Amazon Encore, 2010.

Negron, Ray. **The Boy of Steel: A Baseball Dream Come True.** Michael has brain cancer. But when Yankee second baseman Robinson Cano visits Michael in the hospital, Michael becomes a Yankee batboy for a day. Regan, 2006.

Rapp, Adam. **Punkzilla.** Punkzilla is on a mission to see his older brother "P", before "P" dies of cancer. Still buzzing from his last hit of meth, he embarks on a day's-long trip from Portland, Ore. to Memphis, Tenn., writing letters to his family and friends. Along the way, he sees a sketchier side of America and worries if he will make it to see his brother in time. Candlewick Press, 2009.

Schultz, Charles M. **Why, Charlie Brown, Why?** When Linus's friend develops leukemia, questions arise that are answered here in words, conversations and pictures. Ballantine Books, 2002.

Sonnenblick , Jordan. **After Ever After.** Jeffrey is a teen in remission. Even though the cancer should be far behind him, Jeffrey still worries that it will return. He has got normal teen stuff to deal with, too. Scholastic Press, 2010.

Stork, Francisco X. **The Last Summer Of The Death Warriors.** Pancho is planning a murder when he is assigned to help D.Q., whose brain cancer has slowed neither his spirit nor his mouth. D.Q. tells Pancho all about his "Death Warrior's Manifesto," which will help him to live out his last days fully. Arthur A. Levine Books, 2010.

REFERENCE
Kellerman, Jonathan. **Psychological aspects of childhood cancer.** An overview of the psychological problems that face children with cancer for professionals and parents. C. C. Thomas, 1980.

Mukherjee, Siddhartha. **Emperor of All Maladies: A Biography of Cancer.** A cellular biologist chronicles cancer from its first documented appearances thousands of years ago through the epic battles in the twentieth century to cure, control, and conquer it to a radical new understanding of its essence. Scribner, 2010.

About Benjamin Rubenstein

Benjamin Rubenstein, author of *TWICE: How I Became A Cancer-Slaying Super Man Before I Turned 21,* was a happy-go-lucky 16-year-old in the Washington DC suburbs when his hip began to hurt. A serious tennis player, a star student, the only kid in his class with a car and the darling of some very cute girls, Benjamin had everything going for him. But he found out fast that his pain was coming from a rare form of cancer – Ewing's sarcoma – that attacks growing boys. He spent the next year at the National Institutes of Health where every tactic of modern medicine was applied to save his life. It worked. Ben won his first battle with cancer.

Winning was always on Benjamin Rubenstein's mind. After he beat cancer, he did not keep up with the kids he had met during his treatment at NIH. Benjamin believed that he was no Sick Kid but a super-powered hero who had a unique ability to withstand the toxic chemicals of cancer therapy and preserve his healthy cells while zapping the round-celled malignancy that had invaded his body. Benjamin did not identify with cancer victims. He was a winner, and he continued the fight alone. He went on to the University of Virginia despite losing a year of high school to cancer treatment.

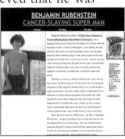

An excerpt from Benjamin Rubenstein's website, Cancer-Slaying Super Man

Then, the most common of blood tests – the CBC, or Complete Blood Count – changed everything. It showed that his bone marrow was dying without his even knowing it. Ben was already mentally preparing himself for going to battle with his second severe illness. He was the self-proclaimed Greatest Cancer Patient Ever and had to live up to his reputation. And for the second time, he did. Benjamin survived cancer. Twice.

READ MORE from Benjamin Rubenstein's website, "Cancer-Slaying Super Man," at www.benjaminrubenstein.com

READ BENJAMIN RUBENSTEIN'S BLOG

DANCING WITH FEAR: A DAY IN MY LIFE WITHOUT A LEFT PELVIC BONE

THURSDAY, JUNE 13, 2013

I walk like a penguin, I think, chuckling at my short stride. The pain in my hip is significant when I shift weight to my left leg. The pain ascends rapidly the further I step forward, so I shuffle. This sensation is not deep inside like the lightning strikes I felt when my tumor was growing long ago, but instead it shoots out towards my abductors. I envision my pain as an iron plate, compacted by the burden of cancer, consuming the space formerly occupied by cancerous bone. This plate does not

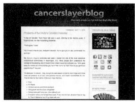

Excerpted from Benjamin
Rubenstein's "Cancer Slayer Blog"
Thursday, June 13, 2013

respect my orthopedic oncology surgeon's handiwork – muscle stapled and taped to other muscle – and is waiting to explode downward, like it is playing Don't Break the Ice against my soft tissue. I think back on recent events to uncover the pain's cause...

READ MORE from Benjamin Rubenstein's "Cancer Slayer Blog" at www.cancerslayerblog.com

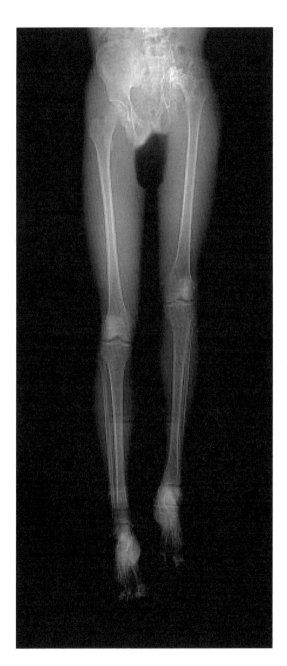

Ewing's sarcoma is a form of bone cancer that frequently appears in the pelvis or long bone of the thigh. It is more common in teenage boys than girls.

You will also want to read TWICE

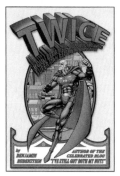

Teenager Benjamin Rubenstein, author of *TWICE: How I Became A Cancer-Slaying Super Man Before I Turned 21*, went through a year of harrowing treatment at the National Institutes of Health after he developed Ewing's sarcoma. He survived, only to be struck down by cancer again at 19 while attending the University of Virginia. After another round of treatment, this time at the University of Minnesota, he survived again.

To endure such fear and pain not once but twice, Benjamin Rubenstein, like Clark Kent, had to develop an alter ego. This device of the cancer-slaying Superman, drawing on the comic book hero's Jewish roots, enabled Benjamin Rubenstein to set aside self-pity and focus on the annihilation of the round cells that were attacking his body.

Like many bright boys of his generation, Benjamin Rubenstein embraces genetics, probability, pharmacology and psychology with a sophistication that was unknown to earlier generations of cancer survivors. The spiritual solace to cancer sufferers in middle age was not available to a young man like Benjamin Rubenstein. The ironic optimism expressed in so many cancer memoirs was lost on him. All he had was an athlete's single-mindedness and the quantitative skills he was learning as an engineering student to bring him to remission. At the dawn of his adult life, Benjamin Rubenstein was not about to be struck down by the disease of "men when they retire." He doesn't try to figure out why he got sick or what he did wrong. Instead, his hospital odyssey challenges this habit of thought in a text that is daring, detailed and impudent.

TWICE How I Became A Cancer-Slaying Super Man Before I Turned 21
(ISBN: 978-0-9786472-9-2) is available at WoodleyBooks.com for $32.00

About the typeface

The text of this book is set in Bembo,
Created in 15th century Venice by
Francesco Griffo for the scholar Pietro Bembo.
Under the direction of Stanley Morison,
Bembo was redesigned in 1929
For the Monotype Typeface Corporation.

This typeface references old style type designs
While adding calligraphic features, resulting in a face
That blends classic proportions with the warmth
Of handwriting.

This popular typeface is sometimes used for
Advertising and display purposes, but,
As seen here, it has the legibility to be useful
In long type settings as well.